About the Author

Roy Upton, a professional herbalist for the past 18 years, is trained in both Western and traditional Chinese herbal medicine. He is the founder and executive director of the American Herbal Pharmacopoeia, an educational organization dedicated to the development of authoritative monographs on botanical medicine; a founding member and vice president of the American Herbalists Guild; and a member of the American Herbal Products Association Standards Committee, a trade organization devoted to establishing quality control standards for herbal supplements.

Mr. Upton was the managing editor and co-author of a monograph on St. John's wort recently published by the American Botanical Council that is considered the most comprehensive technical review of this herb in English. He is also the author of *Echinacea,* another title in the Keats Good Herb Guide series.

Nature's Premier Antidepressant

St. John's wort is the most well-researched of all the antidepressant herbs. In August 1996, the prestigious *British Medical Journal* published a landmark article on the benefits of this common herb for the treatment of mild to moderate depression. For the 18 million Americans suffering from depression, this was good news indeed, since St. John's wort carries none of the unpleasant side effects of conventional antidepressant medications, and it is much less expensive.

This versatile herb has other uses as well. It is considered among the most efficacious wound-healing balms of all botanicals, a wonderful remedy to have on hand for scrapes, sprains, burns and bruises. It is also helpful in treating many types of neuralgic disorders, including sciatica, general nerve pain, carpal tunnel syndrome, shingles and even bedwetting in children.

A KEATS GOOD HERB GUIDE

MEDICINE FOR THE 21ST CENTURY

ST. JOHN'S WORT

The premier herb for relieving depression, healing wounds and easing nerve pain

Roy Upton

Keats Publishing, Inc. New Canaan, Connecticut

St. John's Wort is not intended as medical advice. It's intent is solely informational and educational. Please consult a health professional should the need for one be indicated.

ST. JOHN'S WORT

Library of Congress Cataloging-in-Publication Data

Upton, Roy
St. John's wort / Roy Upton.
p. cm. – (Keats good herb guide)
Includes bibliographical references and index.
ISBN 0-87983-813-2
1. Depression, Mental – Alternative treatment.
2. Hypericum perforatum – Therapeutic use. I. Title. II. Series.
RC537.U68 1997
616.8'527061 – dc21 97-36800
CIP

Printed in the United States of America

Good Herb Guides are published by
Keats Publishing, Inc.
27 Pine Street (Box 876)
New Canaan, Connecticut 06840-0876
Website address: www.keats.com

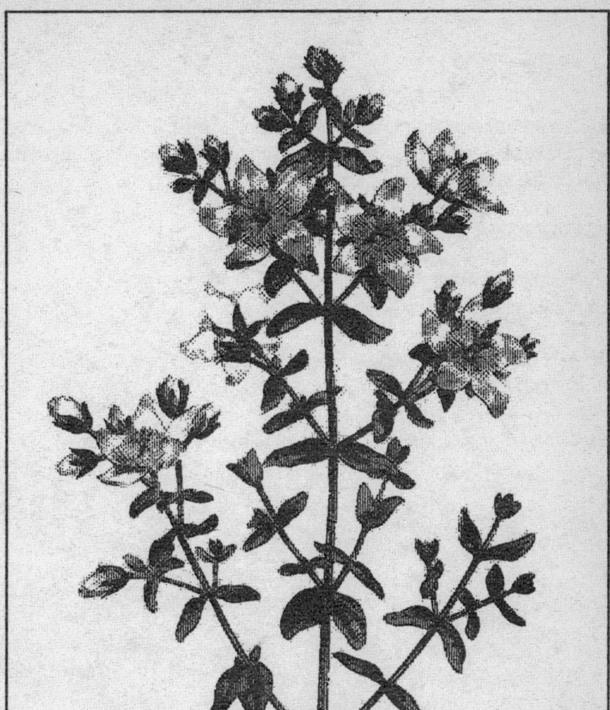

St. John's Wort (*Hypericum perforatum*)

From: *Woodville's Medical Botany*, 3rd ed., 1832

Contents

Introduction

> *"So then about her brow they bound* Hypericum, *whose potent leaves have sovereign power o'er all the sullen fits and cheerless fancies that besiege the mind; banishing ever, to their native night, dark thoughts, and causing to spring up within the heart distress'd a glow of gladdening hope, and rainbow visions of kind destiny."*
>
> —ALFRED LEAR HUXFORD, 1853

The short writing above colorfully illustrates the historical use of St. John's wort *(Hypericum perforatum)* for the treatment of mental and emotional imbalances. In fact, St. John's wort, perhaps more than any other herb, has been used throughout the centuries for various forms of depression, melancholy and sadness as well as for numerous other purposes including wound-healing.

In August of 1996, the *British Medical Journal* published a landmark article on the benefits of St. John's wort for the treatment of mild to moderate depression. This stimulated a tremendous amount of media interest in the herb, culminating in the summer of 1997 with an ABC 20/20 feature presentation that interviewer Barbara Walters called "one of the most important stories we have done for years." For the 18 million

Americans suffering from depression every year, learning about the benefits of St. John's wort may be one of the most important lessons of their lives. What is more, if any of the early clinical trials being conducted regarding its potential as an antiviral agent against AIDS are promising, perhaps there will be more media attention to follow.

The Colorful History of St. John's Wort

St. John's wort has been used in herbal medicine for at least 1,400 years. Throughout its long and colorful history, it has remained one of the most widely used botanicals for the treatment of diseases which would today be classified as mental illness.

In ancient times, St. John's wort served as an amulet to ward off demons and to treat possession. There are several stories of how St. John's wort got its name. One of the earliest recorded accounts is found in a Gaelic legend dating from approximately the sixth century A.D. which stated that the missionary St. Columbia always carried a piece of *Hypericum* in honor of St. John the Baptist, who was said to be fond of the herb.[1] In England there was a tradition of throwing St. John's wort into a bonfire on the eve of St. John's day (June 23). In another account it is reported that early Christians believed that red spots, which they symbolically attributed to the blood of St. John, appeared on the leaves on August 29, the anniversary of St. John's beheading. Another association of the herb with the saint is due to the fact that in many climates, the optimum time to pick St. John's wort is in the middle of summer, around St. John's day. Perhaps the most interesting explanation for the herb's name is that its fresh yellow flowers and buds, when bruised, exude a red pigment that was also symbolically referred to as the blood of St. John.

Other religious nomenclature has been assigned to St. John's wort which attests to the high regard various cultures had for it. This included the Irish *allus Muire* (Mary's sweat), *lus ra Maighdine Muire* (Virgin Mary's herb) and the Welsh name *Creu-lys bendiged* (the blessed herb of an earnest cry or prayer).[2]

St. John's wort was also commonly known as "balm of warrior's wound" because of its widespread use as a primary wound-healing (vulnerary) herb.[1] The name "wort" is a term that was applied to numerous medicinal plants.

The Latin binomial *Hypericum perforatum* is no less interesting and meaningful. Hypericum is derived from the Greek word root *hyper* meaning "above" or "over" and *eikon* meaning "image." This relates back to a European practice of hanging St. John's wort over religious objects. Perforatum comes from *perforatus* which means "pores," referring to the numerous translucid oil glands that are observed when a leaf of the herb is held up to light. Because the herb was often used to help get rid of "evil spirits" and to release one from demonic possession it was also called the *Fuga Demonum* (the Devil's Scourge).

> *St. John's wort doth charm all the witches away, if gathered at midnight on the saint's holy day. And devils and witches have no power to harm those that do gather the plant for a charm; rub the lintels and post with that red juicy flower; no thunder nor tempest will then have the power to hurt or to hinder your houses; and bind round your neck a charm of a similar kind.*
>
> –RAVEN
> Folklore of Staffordshire

Ancient Medical Uses

One of the earliest authorities on herbal medicine was Pedannius Dioscorides, who lived in the first century A.D. He is one of the most noted medical botanists of all time; and, one of the most highly trained medical professionals of his day. His works remained among the most authoritative discourses on medicine for centuries. Dioscorides was born in Anazarbus along the Pyramus river in the former Roman province Cilicia which is now Turkey. In the introduction to his most significant work, *De Materia Medica*, Dioscorides reveals that he took a particular interest in medicinal substances at an early age and was inspired to study drugs by Areios of Tarsus, a medical writer on pharmacy. At the time, Tarsus was an intellectual center that surpassed even Athens and Alexandria and, in particular, was a center of study for pharmacy and pharmacology, as reported by noted medical historian John Riddle. Dioscorides goes on to write that he traveled widely, living a "soldier-like" life dedicated to the study of medicinal plants. His writings also cite numerous provinces and habitats from Greece to Egypt where the plants grew. One key point that Dioscorides personally reports is that his work was based on his own experience and experimentation, rather than simply relying on the findings recorded by his predecessors.

Dioscorides reported on the use of four different species of *Hypericum* for the treatment of sciatica. For this use, he mentions a specific preparation of St. John's wort mixed with water and honey. St. John's wort was one of only ten herbs recommended by Dioscorides for the treatment of wounds, most specifically, burns. He further reports that the herb was used as a diuretic, to move the menses and to allay malarial-type fevers.[3,4]

Other authoritative ancient writers such as Theophrastus, Hippocrates, Pliny and Galen all reported on the medicinal uses of a variety of *Hypericum* species plants for both internal and topical use. Today, St. John's wort's antidepressant effects tend to overshadow its many other therapeutic uses. Among these are its ability to treat bedwetting in children, its usefulness in a myriad of neuralgic complaints such as carpal tunnel syndrome, sciatica and shingles, its primary use as one of the most valued wound-healing herbs throughout the centuries and its more recent use as a potential antiviral in the management and treatment of AIDS.

DOCTRINE OF SIGNATURES

During the Middle Ages and perhaps even before, it was very common for people to ascertain the use of a plant according to its physical characteristics. For example, the herb lung wort *(Pulmonaria lobata)* was thought to resemble a diseased lung, and was therefore assumed to be able to heal a diseased lung. This approach was known as the Doctrine of Signatures. While the Doctrine of Signatures has never been accepted within the world of science, it was traditionally utilized as a training tool among folk herbalists for teaching and building general societal knowledge about the medicinal uses of plants. Over time, those herbs whose activity corresponded with the physical characteristics ascribed to them through the Doctrine of Signatures were remembered and passed down through written and oral tradition, providing us with the basis of much of our herbal medicine today.

John Cole, England's foremost exponent of the Doctrine of Signatures, noted that the little holes (glands) in the leaves of St. John's wort resembled the pores of the skin and divined that this plant could thus be used for skin problems, including bleeding and bruising,[2] a use that has been substantiated through modern experience and experimentation. Another renowned man of medicine who relied on the Doctrine of Signatures was Nicholas Culpeper (1649). An extremely influential and controversial figure in medical history, Culpeper's greatest contribution to medicine was his English translation of the *Pharmacopoeia Londinensis*. Up until that time, the pharmacopoeia was reserved for the elite medical community and was only available in Latin. Culpeper believed that medical knowledge should be shared with common people, however, and was therefore largely ostracized for challenging the medical hierarchy. Culpeper was also an astrologer who assigned planetary associations to plants. St. John's wort was under the dominion of the sun, Culpeper reported, perhaps divining the photoreactivity that can occur when toxic amounts of St. John's wort are consumed.

Introduction of St. John's Wort in the United States

St. John's wort was brought to the United States by European settlers. As St. John's wort was not widely used for other purposes, except perhaps as a dye, it can be presumed that its primary value was medicinal. One of the earliest reports of its domestic use was noted in the late 1700s by Jean-Bernard Bossu, who wrote of the local Louisiana practice of using of St. John's wort oil for healing wounds.

Use of St. John's Wort by the Eclectics

St. John's wort was also used in the 1800s by a group of American physicians known as the eclectics. At that time, there were various schools of medical thought. The predecessors of today's physicians were known as "mineral doctors" because of their reliance on mineral drugs such as mercury compounds (calomel). Today such doctors are referred to as "allopathic physicians." The other primary therapies utilized by the mineral doctors were bleeding and scarification. In contrast, the eclectics relied predominantly on botanically derived medicines, steadfastly denouncing what they considered to be the barbaric bleeding and purging therapies of the mineral doctors. The eclectics amassed a great deal of clinical knowledge and experience in Western herbal medicine that is still relied upon today.

One of the most highly respected of all the eclectic physicians was John "Pappy" King. Dr. King's text, the *American Dispensatory,* remains one of the most valued texts of modern medical herbalists. In the 1898 edition of King's text, St. John's wort is reported to be used as an astringent, diuretic and sedative for the treatment of chronic urinary conditions, diarrhea, dysentery, jaundice, worms, painful menstruation, nervous conditions associated with depression and hemorrhage. The book also states that St. John's wort has a specific effect on the spinal cord; this has led many herbalists to utilize it for a variety of complaints associated with the nervous system including neuralgic pain.

Since its introduction to the U.S., St. John's wort has spread, growing prolifically in pastures and along riverbeds. However, it has become the bane of cattlemen, as cattle who consume large amounts of it develop symptoms of photosensitivity resulting in dermatitis, rapid heartbeat and respiration, and diarrhea. Great lengths have been taken to eradicate the herb. One drastic measure, which has resulted in a significant decrease in naturalized populations, was the introduction in 1946 of the Australian flea beetle *(Chrysolina quadrigemina)*, observed to have a voracious appetite for St. John's wort. The beetle was so successful that it was reported that by 1957 northern California stands of St. John's wort were reduced to only 1 percent of their original numbers.[3] The fact that the herb has become a nuisance to cattlemen is ironic as historically the growing of St. John's wort among cattle was considered a sign the herd would prosper throughout the year.[2]

> *St. John's wort, St. John's wort. My envy whosoever has thee. I will pluck thee with my right hand. I will preserve thee with my left hand. Whoso findeth thee in the cattle-fold. Shall never be without kine.*
>
> Gaelic incantation
> ALEXANDER CARMICHAEL, 1832-1912

Official eradication programs continue here and in other countries. This may eventually lead to the decimation of this valuable medicine.

THE EUROPEAN EXPERIENCE

Europe has a long history of using herbs as an integral part of health care. In most European countries it is legally required that an herbal product disclose its use on its label. However, current regulatory restraints prevent Americans from having access to this information on a product label. In Europe, not only are medicinal herbs allowed and required to carry the appropriate therapeutic information; in many European nations such as Germany and France their use is reimbursed under the national healthcare system. Herbal medicines are similarly covered under the healthcare systems of China, India and Japan. As Americans, we may feel we have access to the best system of medicine available; however, when it comes to herbal medicine, we are incredibly far behind almost all other developed and developing nations.

St. John's wort has been a staple of European herbalism for centuries. It is very common for households to have a St. John's wort ointment or oil on hand as a household remedy. In recent years, St. John's wort has become the most relied upon of all antidepressants throughout Europe. Approximately 66 million doses of St. John's wort are consumed every day in Germany. As an antidepressant, it out-sells Prozac by a factor of 20 to one and out-sells all other antidepressants combined. Its widespread use in Europe has stimulated growing interest in the herb in the United States.

Modern Uses of St. John's Wort

Chemistry of St. John's Wort

There are numerous compounds within St. John's wort that have stimulated interest among medical researchers. The most notable of these are classes of constituents known as napthodianthrones, flavonoids, xanthones and phloroglucinols. See Appendix (page 55) for diagrams of the chemical constituents. The napthodianthrones consist predominantly of two compounds known as hypericin and pseudohypericin. These are the red pigments responsible for the color observed when the herb's flowers are bruised. Other constituents considered equally or even more important than the napthodianthrones are a wide variety of flavonoids contained in both the leaves and flowers. Flavonoids are a class of compounds that are essential to human health and exhibit a wide variety of biological activities.

Activity of Constituents of St. John's Wort	
Constituent	**Activity**
Napthodianthrones: Hypericin, pseudohypericin	Antiviral, MAO inhibitor (in vitro), photodynamic[24, 25, 26]
Flavonoids: Amentoflavone (I3,II8-biapigenin), catechin, epicatechin, hyperoside, kaempferol, luteolin, myricetin, quercetin, quercitrin, iso-quercitrin, I3,II8-biapigenin, rutin	Anti-inflammatory, antiulcerogenic,[5] antioxidant, antimicrobial, antiviral,[6] enhances coronary blood flow[7]
Phloroglucinols: Hyperforin, adhyperforin	Antibacterial, wound-healing[8]
Phenolic Acids: Caffeic acid, chlorogenic acid, gentistic acid, ferulic acid	Immunostimulating
Essential Oils: Monoterpenes, sesquiterpenes	Antibacterial

DEPRESSION IN AMERICA

Seventeen percent of all Americans can expect to suffer from some type of clinical depressive disorder in their lifetime, with women being two times more likely to experience depression than men. Depression does not appear to preferentially affect people of different races, and it is a significant problem among adolescents.

There is no definitive cause of depression. It, of course, affects all of us to some extent at some time in our lives and is a natural response to specific situations such as loss of a loved one or being diagnosed with a life-threatening disease. However, when it affects our life on a daily long-term basis or becomes incapacitating and it matches specific clinical criteria established by various organizations such as the National Institutes of Health, then it becomes a clinically diagnosable disease.

There are two primary types of depression: major depression and dysthymia or chronic low-grade depression. The primary characteristic associated with major depression is that it incapacitates individuals so they are not able to work or sometimes cannot even get out of bed. In addition they may experience symptoms such as insomnia, fatigue, anxiety, feelings of guilt, inability to concentrate or thoughts of suicide. The symptoms usually represent a deviation from the person's normal state of well-being and have persisted for at least two weeks. Chronic depression, on the other hand, occurs over a period of at least two years, with no two consecutive months when the person has been depression-free. In addition, at least two other symptoms such as insominia, anxiety or fatigue must be present. Manic-depressive (bipolar) disorder, or the vascillation between a state of manic high spirits and depression, is also very common. However, St. John's wort has not yet been reported to be helpful for this disorder.

It is estimated that 95 percent of those diagnosed with depression suffer from fatigue and 90 percent experience some level of anxiety. Two-thirds of depressed patients contemplate suicide while approximately 10 to 15 percent will attempt suicide. When depression goes untreated, it is estimated to last from 6 to 13 months; when treated, approximately 3 months.

Depression is in part a consequence of abnormal brain functioning. Normal brain function, and subsequently, behavioral and emotional well-being, is dependent upon the presence of specific chemicals (neurotransmitters) which are responsible for eliciting normal reactions to stimuli between the brain and our external environment. There are numerous neurotransmitters. Those predominantly associated with depression are collectively known as catecholamines which include epinephrine, norepinephrine, the amino acid Dopa, dopamine and serotonin. Many of the conventional antidepressant medications work by allowing more of these neurotransmitters to be available to the brain by inhibiting the enzymes that break down neurotransmitters or by potentiating the effects of neurotransmitters. These medications include monoamine oxidase (MAO) inhibitors, tricyclic antidepressants (TCAs) and serotonin-specific reuptake inhibitors (SSRIs). Prozac is the most well known of the SSRIs and is currently the third most widely prescribed drug in the United States.

While conventional antidepressants can benefit those suffering from depression, they possess a myriad of negative side effects, many of which in themselves can be debilitating or can, over time, lead to liver damage. One of the key advantages of St. John's wort is that it has been shown to be as effective as many of the conventional antidepressants, but with almost no side effects.

ST. JOHN'S WORT AS A MAO INHIBITOR

Interest in St. John's wort among medicinal plant researchers was initially stimulated by studies reporting that St. John's wort was an effective MAO inhibitor. This finding was later reported in the St. John's wort German Commission E monograph which described its use for the treatment of psychogenic disturbances, depressive states, anxiety or nervous excitement based on its presumed function as a MAO inhibitor. This contributed to the widespread use of St. John's wort among German clinicians for the treatment of various types of depression and helped to stimulate continued interest among researchers in articulating its mechanisms of action, an endeavor which has yet to be definitive.

Much debate has taken place as to whether St. John's wort is an effective MAO inhibitor. In a 1981 study, researchers reported on the ability of a class of plant-derived compounds known as xanthones to strongly inhibit the monoamine oxidases *in vitro*.[9] Xanthones are commonly found in members of the *Guttiferae* family to which St. John's wort belongs. A 1994 study reported similar findings suggesting that one species of St. John's wort, *Hypericum brasiliense*, yielded xanthones that had a significant MAO-inhibiting effect.[10] However, xanthones are predominantly found in the roots of *Hypericum* plants. In European and American herbal medicine the flowering tops and leaves are predominantly used medicinally, not the roots.

Acknowledging the long history of use of St. John's wort as an antidepressant in a subsequent study, the first group of researchers, Suzuki, et al., investigated the MAO-inhibitory effects of one of St. John's wort's primary components, the napthodianthrone hypericin. Hypericin is a pigment which is partially responsible for the red coloring that exudes from the herb's fresh flowers when they are bruised. The researchers reported that hypericin inhibited both MAO_A and MAO_B in *in vitro* studies.[11] However, the subsequent researchers, Rocha, et al., reported more potent MAO-inhibitory effects with the xanthones[10] while still others reported more significant MAO-inhibiting activity associated with specific flavonoids.[12, 13, 14] In addition, the molecular structures of various components of St. John's wort were compared with known MAO inhibitors. In this report, only specific flavones were considered similar enough to potentially act as MAO inhibitors.[15]

These studies in part established the theory that the primary mode of St. John's wort's antidepressant activity was via MAO inhibition. However, while other researchers corroborated the MAO-inhibiting activity of various *Hypericum* constituents and crude extracts, the dosage required to achieve this effect was many times greater than could be achieved with standard St. John's wort preparations that were proven, effective antidepressants. Therefore, most researchers who have reviewed the data recently conclude that a wide variety of constituents and mechanisms of action other than MAO inhibition must be responsible for the antidepressant activity of St. John's wort.[12, 14, 16]

Other potential mechanisms of action have been put forth including St. John's wort's potential as a catecholamine-O-methyltransferase (COMT) inhibitor.[16] Like MAO inhibitors, COMT inhibitors interfere with the enzyme that breaks down catecholamines, allowing more to be available to the brain. COMT inhibition has been demonstrated with the use of St. John's wort alcohol extracts, and again this activity was attributed to the flavonoids and occurred at high dosages. Other proposed mechanisms are its potential to inhibit serotonin receptor expression, the inhibition of serotonin reuptake, inhibition of GABA uptake and an inhibition of cytokine expression. The first three activities, as with MAO inhibition, have only occurred at dosages far greater than are obtainable from the crude extracts used; therefore they are insufficient to explain St. John's wort's activity. The fourth activity (inhibition of cytokine expression) is equally undefinitive.[17]

A novel mechanism that has recently been suggested is that St. John's wort may have an effect on melatonin activity and production. Melatonin, the principal hormone produced by the pineal gland, plays an important role in behavior and sleep. The pineal gland was called the "seat of the soul" by the philosopher Descartes and was for a long time considered the remnant of a "third eye" high in the back of the head in animals. It plays a primary role in the regulation of sexual and reproductive function and also has a role in promoting deep sleep. Many other functions have been associated with melatonin, including the ability to mitigate symptoms associated with jet lag as well as antioxidant activities. In addition, melatonin has also been shown to reduce anxiety-like behavior in animals.[18]

It has been theorized that St. John's wort may increase the efficacy of retinal mechanisms that can transform light impulses into neuronal signals, which can in turn modulate the internal production and utilization of endogenously produced melatonin. St. John's wort also was reported to contribute to a slight increase in melatonin production.[19] St. John's wort has a long history as a sleep aid, especially in sleeplessness associated with fear and anxiety, which is similar to the activity reported for melatonin. Further study in this area is needed.

ST. JOHN'S WORT BLOSSOMS IN AMERICA

As mentioned earlier, increased interest in St. John's wort in America was stimulated by a published article in the prestigious *British Medical Journal (BMJ)* (Aug. 1996). St. John's wort has long been a staple of American herbalism, predominantly for its external use in the treatment of scrapes, burns and abrasions and secondarily for pains of neuralgic origin. Its antidepressant effects, though known by some herbalists, went largely unheralded until recently. Early German articles and the 1996 BMJ study changed this. Almost immediately, reports of its effectiveness were picked up by the Ameican popular media. Word got out that St. John's wort was safer than and just as effective as conventional antidepressants, it was relatively inexpensive, and it outsold Prozac in Germany by a factor of approximately 20 to 1. Immediately, St. John's wort products began appearing and disappearing off of the shelves as fast as clerks and pharmacists could unpack the boxes, quickly depleting the herb's supply pipelines, which predominantly originate in Europe.

On the 20/20 TV presentation, Dr. Harold Bloomfield, a Yale-trained psychiatrist, reported having recommended St. John's wort for several hundred patients, from which he based his conclusion that St. John's wort is the first therapy to try in the majority of depressive disorders. While the majority of the clinical studies conducted with St. John's wort were of short duration, the few patients interviewed on this presentation had been using St. John's wort with positive results for six months to one year. Dr. Bloomfield went on to predict that St. John's wort just might become America's leading antidepressant.

Clinical Studies

In the 1996 *BMJ* article, 23 randomized trials were reviewed, which included 1,757 patients with mild to moderately severe depression. The authors concluded that *Hypericum* extracts were significantly superior to a placebo and as effective as standard depressants. Moreover, those patients using St. John's wort experienced significantly fewer side effects than those using standard medications.

Many studies have shown St. John's wort to be superior to a placebo. At least 18 controlled studies have compared it with the conventional antidepressant imipramine, with many researchers concluding that it is as effective as this standard medication. In one randomized double-blind study, St. John's wort was compared to another conventional antidepressant, maprotiline. A total of 102 patients were diagnosed with moderately severe depression according to international classification scales* and then administered either the maprotiline or the St. John's wort preparation (LI 160). In a four-week period, similar improvements were observed with both substances.[20] Maprotiline was slightly more effective than the St. John's wort preparation as an antidepressant when assessed according to two of the scales, but the patients using St. John's wort and assessed according to the Clinical Global Impression scale reported a greater feeling of well-being than those taking

* ICD-10, F 32.1. Patients who have experienced a single, moderately severe depressive episode accompanied by a general depressive state, lack of interest and happiness, and reduction in motivation; the Hamilton Depression Scale; Depression scale according to von Zerssen and the Clinical Global Impression Scale.

maprotiline. In addition, there were fewer side effects reported for St. John's wort than for maprotiline.

In another review of 3,250 patients (49 percent with mild depression, 46 percent with intermediate depression, 3 percent with severe depression) improvement was observed in 80 percent of the patients taking St. John's wort. Some of the symptoms which were alleviated were sleep disturbances or restlessness, headaches, cardiac irregularities and sweating.[21]

In a study of 105 mildly depressed patients, significant improvement was seen in those treated with St. John's wort as compared to a placebo. Most significant in this study were marked improvements in feelings of sadness, hopelessness, helplessness, worthlessness, difficulty initiating sleep and psychological anxiety. In addition, other subjective symptoms such as sleep disorders, headaches, cardiac symptoms and exhaustion were improved in those using St. John's wort.[22]

At the time of this writing, the National Institutes of Health have issued a request for grant proposals to further study the effectiveness of St. John's wort as an antidepressant. The currently available studies suggest that St. John's wort, as Dr. Bloomfield states, "deserves to be a first line of treatment" for depression. The fact that it appears to be as effective as standard medications and that very few side effects have been reported in the tens of thousands of patients using it makes it an ideal choice before resorting to the more powerful, expensive and potentially toxic standard antidepressants.

Despite all of the positive data on the benefits of St. John's wort, there are still those who caution against its use either because an exact mechanism of action is not known or because most of the trials conducted to date were of relatively short duration. However, equally undefinitive and limited scientific data are available to confirm the safety and effectiveness of the majority of conventional antidepressant medications currently being prescribed. We have 20 or so years of experience with conventional medications in contrast to 1,400 years of experience using St. John's wort. When all is said and done, it would appear that St. John's wort should be the first therapeutic agent to be tried by those suffering from depression. See the Appendix for a summary chart of the clinical studies.

Comprehensive St. John's Wort Antidepressant Program

Many ill people want magic bullet cures. They want to ease their discomfort simply by swallowing a pill or liquid with little fuss or involvement. Unfortunately, this is how many of us have been conditioned because of the "miracles" of conventional medicine. Our parents, schools and physicians do not teach us how to take care of ourselves through diet, lifestyle modifications, nutritional supplements and herbs. Instead, we are taught simply to swallow a pill. However, this is not effective self-care. To be truly healthy requires self-knowledge, a certain level of discipline, persistence, and in some cases, hard work.

Any medicine or herb should be used only within the context of a health-promoting lifestyle that encompasses proper diet, exercise, stress reduction and sufficient rest. This is especially true when using St. John's wort for the management and treatment of a depressive or psychological disorder. A few components of a comprehensive antidepressant program using St. John's wort follow.

Counseling: One of the most important aspects of a comprehensive treatment program for depression is counseling. There are two primary forms: psychoanalysis and cognitive/behavioral therapy. The primary goal of psychoanalysis is to heal past emotional wounds that may be a source of unconscious anger, frustration, guilt or shame that can contribute to depressive disorders. Pscychoanalysis reasons that if the emotional wounds of the past are not acknowledged or appropriately addressed then the problems of today which are directly caused or exacerbated by them will continue or worsen. Therefore, psychoanalysis tries to help resolve such traumas.

The primary goal of cognitive/behavioral therapy is to replace unhealthy thinking patterns, also known as "cognitive distortions," with healthier thinking patterns. If we become conscious of our thinking, we realize that we all have experienced some level of cognitive distortion at some point in our lives, if not on an everyday basis. The basis of our thinking patterns, good and bad, comes predominantly from our past experiences and conditioning. Our thinking patterns affect every aspect of our lives and influence every decision we make and every personal interaction we have. Therefore, cognitive/behavioral therapy is used to help a patient replace negative thinking patterns with more positive thinking patterns. The type of counseling one seeks should be determined by the individual needs of the client.

In addition to counseling, a comprehensive program should include effective stress reduction techniques (deep breathing exercises, yoga, meditation, positive thinking tapes, prayer, etc.) that one can do on a daily basis on one's own as part of a self-healing program. Also, it is important to develop a support system of good friends and/or family that will provide the reassurance, assistance and love needed to overcome periods of depression.

Diet: Maintaining adequate blood sugar levels and nutritional intake is extremely important, especially in the management and treatment of depression. The energy needs of the brain are greater than all other organs. As blood sugar levels go down, oftentimes the level of emotional well-being similarly declines. This is not because of disease but simply because the brain lacks nourishment and thus cannot perform in an optimal manner; this can manifest as depression.

The two most important dietary principles to follow are to eat sufficient quantities of food for the amount of energy expended on a daily basis, and to assure that the food is of high nutritional value. Overconsumption of white flour and sugared products, refined grains and processed foods will lead to significant nutritional deficiencies and sugar highs and lows that can negatively affect brain chemistry. Regular consumption of complex carbohydrates and proteins such as are found in whole grains, fresh vegetables and legumes, together with relatively smaller amounts of animal protein will help to sustain the steady blood sugar levels that contribute to emotional stability.

Nutritional supplements: There is data supporting the use of specific nutrients to promote mental and emotional well-being in addition to maintaining well-balanced blood sugar levels and sound nutritional integrity through proper diet. These supplements include GABA, tyrosine, l-tryptophane, l-phenylalanine and glutamine. The amino acids tyrosine and l-trytophane are biochemical precursors leading to the production of dopamine. L-phenylalanine is a precursor to phenylethylamine, an endogenously produced antidepressant substance reported to be lacking in depressed patients.[23] Though not strictly a nutritional supplement, the hormone melatonin is also recommended.

Other botanical supplements: There are a few other botanicals noted for their antidepressant effects. These include: Kava kava *(Piper methysticum)*, an herb that has been used in the South Pacific as a ceremonial and social drink, perhaps for centuries. Modern pharmacological research suggests its primary uses are as an antianxiety, anticonvulsant and sleep-inducing agent, while some who use kava report significant mood-elevating effects. Various kava preparations are available on the commercial market.

Lemon balm *(Melissa officinalis)*, which is widely used in Europe, was historically used for "melancholy" and "hysteria" and is currently used as an antianxiety and sleep agent. Like St. John's wort, it is a specific for sleeplessness due to nervous tension. Though lacking the scientific evidence that exists for St. John's wort, it has enjoyed a long history of use as a mood elevator. As Shakespeare wrote, "lemon balm doth make the heart merry."

Reishi mushroom *(Ganoderma lucidum)*, popular in China, is an effective mood-elevating herb that was used by monks in ancient times to promote a calm, centered and focused state of mental well-being. While it does not work specifically as an antidepressant via the mechanisms previously mentioned, it does have specific tonifying properties which very definitely contribute to an improved sense of emotional and mental well-being. Reishi has the added advantage of being one of the most well-researched of all immunomodulating herbs.

Chaste tree berry *(Vitex agnus castus)* is specific for influencing hormonal levels in women. It works via the pituitary gland and can be used for hormonally-induced depressive states such as premenstrual syndrome (PMS) and menopause. Because of its effect on the pituitary, it may also be useful in the treatment of seasonal affective disorder (SAD) which is partly associated with pituitary imbalance, and is a common form of depression in many areas where exposure to sunlight is limited.

Exercise: The human body requires physical activity. Exercise promotes lean muscle mass which can increase energy production. Many times depression is accompanied by physical lethargy. Addressing physical lethargy can often help to decrease mental depression. Another advantage of exercise for mental health is that it produces enkephalins and endorphins, specific mood-elevating neurotransmitters.

Using St. John's Wort with Conventional Medications

Unfortunately, no definitive guidelines are available as to how to incorporate St. John's wort if a patient is already using a standard antidepressant. From the available literature there are no reports of St. John's wort interacting either negatively or positively with other antidepressants. However, as in the treatment of many diseases, switching or adding medications should be done carefully, ideally under the supervision of a qualified health professional. This is especially important for those suffering from severe forms of major depression. Also, one should never discontinue medication too abruptly. With most medications, the body begins to get used to having the substance in its system. If the medication is stopped abruptly, the body may respond dramatically, with the condition being treated becoming worse than before the medication was started. This can last until the body has the chance to readjust to being without the medication. In those contemplating suicide, the consequences can be tragic.

Most important, St. John's wort should be used only where it has been found to be of most benefit–in mild to moderate depressive states. There are very few reports of its usefulness in severe depression, and the risk of having a significant negative reaction with severe depression is high. Even though St. John's wort has not been shown to inhibit MAO in a manner that is of practical relevance, a conservative approach would be not to take St. John's wort along with conventional MAO inhibitors in order to avoid the potential for triggering an additive effect. Similarly, one would not use St. John's wort until two weeks after discontinuing a conventional MAO inhibitor as this kind of medication has a residual effect even after being discontinued. Care should also be taken when using St. John's wort in conjunction with SSRIs as the combination of conventional MAO inhibitors and SSRIs can lead to a significant increase in blood pressure. Any transition from drugs to herbs should be undertaken only under the supervision of a qualified healthcare practitioner.

Additional Uses of St. John's Wort

As mentioner earlier, while the antidepressant effects of St. John's wort have captured the world's attention, this is not the only healing benefit of this wonderful plant. Throughout history, herbalists, physicians and lay people have utilized St. John's wort for a variety of conditions with great success. In addition, a significant amount of scientific study has gone into researching some of its other uses.

Antiviral Activity

German physicians using St. John's wort for the treatment of depression observed that many of their patients experienced a lower incidence of opportunistic infections as compared to the general population. This led to interest in researching St. John's wort for potential antiviral activity. Most of this research has focused on the antiviral effects of two of St. John's wort's primary constituents, the napthodianthrones hypericin and pseudohypericin. Researchers from the New York University Medical Center and the Weizmann Institute of Science in Israel demonstrated that both hypericin and pseudohypericin strongly inhibit a variety of retroviruses, of which HIV is one, *in vitro* and *in vivo*.

A paper published in 1988[24] stated that hypericin and pseudohypericin possessed potent antiretroviral activity. The researchers postulated that these compounds may interfere with viral infection and/or spread of a virus by direct inactivation of the virus or by preventing virus shedding, budding or assembly at the cell membrane. Furthermore, the concentrations of compounds necessary for eliciting an antiviral activity were such that no toxicological concern was evident.

In 1989, a group of Japanese researchers elucidated additional mechanisms responsible for St. John's wort's antiviral activity.[25] They found that both hypericin and pseudohypericin inhibit protein kinase C, which is important in the signal transduction associated with various cellular functions including the proliferation of retroviruses.

In subsequent research it was again found that both hypericin and pseudohypericin were effective antiviral agents against numerous viruses in addition to the human immunodeficiency virus (HIV). These included cytomegalo, herpes simplex 1 and 2, influenza and hepatitis B viruses. It was further noted that the antiviral activity was enhanced upon exposure to light, which elicited St. John's wort's photosensitizing activity.[26] Hypericin was also shown to inhibit the activity of the enzyme succinoxidase, which is thought to be associated with the development of tumors. There have been no long-term clinical AIDS trials in the U.S. although initial trials are now underway. Anecdotal reports of St. John's wort's value for the management of HIV and AIDS is mixed, with some reporting positive findings and others questioning its utility as an antiviral. Many people within the HIV community report on its effectiveness in reducing the incidence of opportunistic infections, promoting an increased feeling of well-being due to its antidepressant effects and increasing energy levels. Substantiated reports of its ability to reduce viral loads in HIV are lacking. However, the herb's ability to reduce the incidence of opportunistic infections in itself is significant, as these infections are one of the most significant problems associated with the decline in health of patients with HIV.

Wound Healing

According to the earliest writings of Western herbal medicine, St. John's wort has been one of the most relied upon wound-healing herbs in the botanical world. Culpeper reported on its use in the treatment of wounds, bruises and bites, even from venomous animals. Another famed herbalist, John Gerard, whose book (a rewrite of an earlier herbal by Parkinson) *The Herbal* (1633) remained the standard text of herbal medicine for more than 200 years, regarded St. John's wort as one of the most highly regarded of vulneraries (wound healers), stating:

> *The leaves, floures and seeds stamped and put into a glass with oyle olive and set in the hot Sunne for certaine weeks together...doth make an oyle the colour of bloud, which is a most precious remedy for deepe wounds and those that are thorow the body, for sinews that are prickt or any wound meade with a venomed weapon.*

In 1891, Anne Pratt, a colorful and prolific English writer, noted that she would collect St. John's wort flowers as a child and that she had much faith in the efficacy of the ointment prepared from them. The eclectics also reported on the herb's use as a fomentation for the treatment of caked breasts, hard tumors and bruising, uses not generally recorded in modern herbals. The eclectics also valued St. John's wort for its wound-healing effects as did early homeopaths.

Homeopaths continue to consider three herbs sovereign in the treatment of traumas. The first of these is arnica, also known as leopard's bane, a beautiful small yellow mountain flower whose oil is specifically used in traumas associated with bruising due to injuries. Arnica can also be taken internally (in minute homeopathic doses, as arnica possesses significant toxicity) for a wide range of physical traumas including the birthing process. The second herb is calendula *(Calendula officinalis)*, the beautiful orange and yellow garden flower, the common pot marigold. An oil, extract or salve is prepared from the dried flowers and is used when tissue has been lacerated as in cuts in order to promote the healing of tissue externally or to facilitate the healing of irritated skin such as diaper rash. Calendula tea or extract is used internally for bleeding ulcers and varicose veins. The third herb homeopaths recommend is St. John's wort, considered the most specific remedy for the tissues of the nervous system–"arnica for the nerves." In addition to those uses already mentioned, the eclectics utilized it for injuries of the spine and in lacerated and puncture wounds to prevent tetanus.

Other types of pains of neuralgic origin are said to respond to both external and internal therapy with St. John's wort. These include inflammation surrounding a painful tooth extraction,[27] herpes zoster and herpes communis, chronic neuralgia originating from fractures, spinal injuries and musculoskeletal or surgical trauma.[17]

There have been a few scientific studies on St. John's wort's wound-healing effects. The compounds considered to be most responsible for this activity are the essential oil, phloroglucinols and flavonoids. In a study in the 1950s, the essential oil and the water-soluble fraction of an alcohol extract were found to exhibit minor antifungal activity and significant antibacterial activity. A resinous fraction was also shown effective against gram-positive and gram-negative organisms.[29] In other studies, the tannins and flavonoids in St. John's wort were reported to inactivate *E. coli*.[30, 31] A different preparation containing quercetin along with St. John's wort was similarly found to be more effective than sulfur antibiotics in the treatment of *Staphylococcus aureus* infection.[32] The phloroglucinols hyperforin and adhyperforin are considered most responsible for many of St. John's wort's healing activities. Both compounds have been reported to possess an antibiotic activity greater than that of sulfonilamide.[32] In one study, a burn ointment prepared from St. John's wort flowers (five grams of flowers to 100 grams olive oil) was used in the treatment of burns. First-degree burns were reported to heal within 48 hours, while second- and third-degree burns healed three times faster than burns treated through conventional means. In addition, the St. John's wort preparation was observed to have an inhibitory action against the development of scar tissue.[33]

In another study, the wound-healing effects of a homeopathic mother tincture (1:10) of St. John's wort was compared with calendula, another widely used wound-healing herb. The effects of St. John's wort administered orally were reported to be greater than that of externally applied calendula tincture. In this study, St. John's wort increased the regeneration of epithelial tissue and the strength and integrity of connective tissue.[34] The oil of St. John's wort is also used clinically for stimulating the healing of compromised and inflamed tissues internally such as in the treatment of gastric ulcer, functional gastritis[35] and inflammatory bowel disease.[36] For gastritis and stomach ulcers, a teaspoon of the oil is taken in the morning and evening. For inflammatory bowel disease, it is reported to be best administered as an overnight retention enema.

Externally, St. John's wort is also used as a fomentation, oil or ointment for bruises, swellings due to trauma and ulcers and is considered a specific in injuries when a considerable amount of peripheral nerve damage has occurred, such as in scrapes and burns. A noted European herbalist, the late Dr. H.C.A. Vogel, provided detailed guidance for various external and internal applications of St. John's wort. One notable use is in the treatment and prevention of varicose veins and phlebitis, especially in pregnancy. For this purpose he recommended that a tea be prepared from a combination of St. John's wort, yarrow and arnica *root* (note that arnica *flowers* possess a significant toxicity and should not be used). He suggested that a compress be prepared from this same tea and wrapped around the varicosities. As an ongoing therapy, Dr. Vogel recommended rubbing the oil over the entire leg once weekly. He added that for phlebitis, relief can be obtained by preparing a compress out of a St. John's wort alcohol extract and wrapping it around the affected area. Similarly, he noted that an ointment of St. John's wort is a specific for treating hemorrhoids. For neuritis, cover the area with the warmed oil, fomentation or compress and cover with a hot water bottle.[37]

A novel use of St. John's wort is the treatment of mumps in children by heating the oil and saturating a cloth with it. The cloth is placed over the affected area and covered with a hot water bottle. This is reported to relieve the pain and discomfort associated with the condition.

In addition to the use of St. John's wort oil to treat various traumas, it has also been widely used to promote healthy skin, and to treat skin conditions such as cradle cap in babies and eczema.

Additional Healing Benefits

Numerous other medicinal benefits of St. John's wort have been largely overlooked because of the focus on its antidepressant and antiviral effects. One of the most common of these is the treatment of bedwetting in children. Though the historical data do not provide any clear guidance in this use, it can presumably be due to St. John's wort's antidepressant effects. The conventional antidepressant imipramine has similarly been found effective in treating enuresis due to psychological reasons.[38]

Another benefit related to the herb's antidepressant activity is its ability to improve the quality of sleep. Historically it has been reported to have sedative qualities, and, additionally, one study mentions its ability to increase deep sleep in a group of elderly patients. However, this study also noted that it did not display a specific sedative action.[39] For the treatment of night-time fears in children, German physician Rudolf Weiss recommends that St. John's wort be combined with herbal sedatives such as hops.

An interesting use of St. John's wort oil reported to be effective is to rub it on areas affected by rheumatic or neuralgic aches or pains. For greater relief, the oiled area may be covered with a towel and then gently pressed with an iron over the area with the iron set on its lowest setting. Obviously, great care has to be taken not to burn oneself. The heat from the iron will thin the oil which will increase local absorption.

St. John's wort oil or ointment can also be used to prevent inflammation of the breasts when breastfeeding. Consistent with historical records and clinical data provided by the eclectics, Dr. Vogel confirms the usefulness of St. John's wort for various conditions associated with the genitourinary tract, including bedwetting in children and bladder infections. For this purpose he recommends combining the herb with calendula and yarrow and making a tea. St. John's wort is also a valuable ingredient in oils used to treat inner ear infections. My favorite combination is a mixture of the oils of St. John's wort, garlic and mullein flowers. After warming the oil, place two to three drops in each ear. This simple therapy can be very effective and can greatly lessen the need for antibiotics, some of which have been found to be worse than no treatment at all.

The *British Herbal Pharmacopoeia* cites St. John's wort as a specific for nervous anxiety due to menopause. For this use it is often combined with the Native American herb black cohosh *(Cimicifuga racemosa)*. In a paper presented at a medicinal plant conference in

Munich, Germany[28] this combination was reported to be beneficial for numerous menopausal symptoms. Hot flashes (77 percent of patients), depression (75 percent of patients), internal strain (67 percent), irritability (64 percent) and concentration disorders disappeared or clearly decreased in severity in 61 percent of patients taking the St. John's wort/black cohosh combination.[28]

Dosage and Use Instructions

Dosages

The most well-defined dosages for St. John's wort are those established for its antidepressant effects. All preparations utilized in the trials cited in the *British Medical Journal* were standardized for hypericin based on the assumption that hypericin is an effective MAO inhibitor. While hypericin appears to be a valuable marker compound for standardizing St. John's wort preparations, it has never been shown to inhibit MAO in tests on humans. As previously noted in this book, the dosage required to inhibit MAO is much higher than can generally be obtained from standard St. John's wort preparations. These limitations aside, the products used in the trials that were reviewed represented a wide range of dosages: between 0.4-2.7 mg of hypericin and from 300 to 1,000 mg of the total extract daily.[40]

Powder:	Two to four grams[41]
Infusion:	One to two teaspoons of herb per cup of water. Drink one to two cups morning and evening.

Tincture:	30 drops three times daily. Reduce to two times daily after four days[38]
Fluid Extract:	Five to 10 drops three times daily.
Oil:	One teaspoon two to three times daily on an empty stomach morning and evening.[36, 38]

The effects of St. John's wort have been reported to be observable within a few days. In several of the studies, positive results were observed within two weeks. Still, other researchers have stated that St. John's wort must be taken for six weeks before positive effects are observed.

SIDE EFFECTS, CONTRAINDICATIONS AND TOXICITY

The toxicology of St. John's wort has been well studied. Most texts report that the herb is a highly toxic compound because of its ability to cause photosensitivity (dermatitis upon exposure to the sun) when large amounts are consumed. Such photosensitivity was first recorded when it was observed that cattle and sheep consuming large amounts of fresh St. John's wort would often develop severe skin problems. This stimulated reports about the herb's toxicology in the scientific literature. However, in clinical trials with more than 3,000 patients, very few side effects were observed, and European pharmacovigilance programs have revealed nothing of significance. While it is possible to experience photosensitivity when consuming St. John's wort, dosages far above the normally recommended clinically effective doses must be consumed. Some references report that the dosage at which side effects are observable is 30 times higher than that recommended to treat depression.[42] Thus far, few side effects have been observed in humans when St. John's wort is consumed within its normal dosage range. However, St. John's wort is reported to have minor uterine-stimulating activity and should therefore not be used during pregnancy.

Since the recent interest in St. John's wort there have been concerns raised about consuming St. John's wort in conjunction with tyramine-containing foods such as cheeses and wines. Such foods are contraindicated for people taking MAO inhibitors. However, as MAO inhibition has not been substantiated with use of St. John's wort in humans or animals, this caution is not considered applicable. Similarly, no such toxicities have been reported in Germany and France, where large amounts of both St. John's wort and tyramine-containing foods are consumed. Concerns regarding the use of St. John's wort in conjunction with conventional antidepressant medications have already been discussed. From a review of the existing literature, no negative interactions with conventional antidepressant drugs should be expected if used with St. John's wort, though it has been shown to potentiate the effects of some barbiturates.[17]

One cautionary note regarding its external use for strains and traumas is important because of St. John's wort's photoreactive potential. When therapists have utilized ultrasound immediately after applying the oil to patients who were subsequently exposed to sunlight, second-degree burns occurred which led to scarring. Thus, St. John's wort oil plus ultrasound plus sunlight is a combination to be avoided.

HARVESTING ST. JOHN'S WORT

There are approximately 370 species of *Hypericum. Hypericum perforatum,* the most widely researched of these species, is native to Europe and all of Asia and has been naturalized in the United States. It grows abundantly throughout the Pacific Northwest, where concerted efforts to eradicate it have taken its toll on naturalized populations. It blooms from June to August and can be found in pastures and hillsides, usually in dry areas with full sunlight.

Hypericum perforatum is the preferred species, though noted North American herbalist Michael Moore reports that the closely related species *Hypericum formosum (Hypericum scouleri)* may also be used, though he considers it to be only half as potent as *H. perforatum.*[43] *H. perforatum* is a shrubby perennial which grows to a height of from two to four feet. The green to pale-green leaves are elliptical to oblong, occurring opposite each other on the stems. A distinguishing characteristic of this species is the leaves' translucent oil glands which are observable when held up to light. The yellow flowers have five petals each and occur in large rounded or flat-topped compound cymes with 25 to 100 flowers each. The flowers often have black dots around the margin of the petals. Another distinguishing characteristic is that the pale green stem is hollow with faint longitudinal opposing ribs. When bruised, the plant has a slightly sweet balsamic aroma and a mildly bitter resinous astringent taste.

St. John's wort should be gathered when blooming on a hot sunny day as the heat causes the essential oils to rise up in the plant. As nighttime comes or on cool overcast days, there are significantly lower amounts of napthodianthrones, flavonoids and phloroglucinols in the top portion of the plant. Once harvested, the material should be protected from light.

Plants should be gathered in areas free from the pollution of automobiles and herbicides. Using a pair of gloves and some clippers makes harvesting easier. Care should be taken to pick only a portion of the top 3 to 6 inches of each individual plant. Harvesting only this portion of the plant yields the highest concentrations of St. John's wort's important constituents and also causes little damage to the herb, enabling the plant to grow back easily. A sampling of each of the plant parts should be gathered including the upper leaves and stems, the buds immediately prior to blooming, the fully opened flowers and the unopened buds if some are present. I prefer to gather a large percentage of unopened buds.

Caution: Care should be taken when harvesting St. John's wort. The filaments of the flowers are very fine and splintery and can get into the eyes, causing contact dermatitis, mucosal irritation and local photosensitivity. Be careful not to touch the face, eyes and mouth when gathering St. John's wort.

Making Your Own Preparations

Bulk material: Dried St. John's wort is available in many stores that specialize in herbs. The material usually consists of a mixture of stems, leaves and flowers. To assure that the material is the correct species, check the stem to see that it has two opposing rib lines. This is a unique characteristic of *Hypericum perforatum.* Usually, the top 12 to 24 inches are gathered, but this is not easily ascertainable as the material is often cut up. There should be a large percentage of leaves and flowers. The leaves should be a deep green, and the yellow color of the flower petals should be noticeable. The herb should have a balsamic odor and an astringent balsamic taste. Oftentimes, the material is cut and sifted so that it is largely unrecognizable. However, the yellow of the flowers should still be apparent. If the material appears to have lost its deep green coloring and the flower petals are brown, the herb is of poor quality.

Infusions (teas): Infusions are prepared by pouring one cup of boiled water over two teaspoons of the dried or fresh herb. Steep for 10 minutes and strain.

Alcohol extracts: When preparing the alcohol extract, most herbalists feel that fresh herb is best, although some research reports that the dried flowers yield the highest amount of constituents. The flowers are extremely delicate, and strict care must be taken to assure the constituents are not destroyed in the drying process. If drying is desired, freeze-drying or drying at 158°F for 10 hours has been reported to preserve the highest level of constituents.[17] A general recommendation is to prepare the extract using 20 grams of herb per 100 ml of extracting solution (alcohol, usually vodka, and water with a finished alcohol concentration of approxmately 70 percent).

To make the extract, place the herb in a blender. Cover with the menstruum (70 percent alcohol). Blend just long enough to thoroughly purée it. This will break down the fibrous material of the leaves and stems, resulting in a greater extracting efficiency. Pour into a mason jar and let stand for two weeks in a dark cool place, shaking the solution every day. Strain off and press through cheesecloth at the end of two weeks. Then strain through a coffee filter to eliminate fine particles. Store in a glass amber bottle, making sure to label it with the name of the plant and the date it was poured off. The expressed liquid should be deep red in color, reminiscent of a good burgundy wine. It should have a resinous and astringent, somewhat balsamic flavor. This product should be good for up to two years.

Oil macerates: Oil preparations are among the most versatile to use on an ongoing basis for minor scrapes and burns and are also valuable for internal use as described earlier. The plant should be harvested in much the same manner as when making alcohol extracts. However, you may want to gather the St. John's wort a little bit later in the year when the seed capsules are maturing. The capsules yield a high concentration of phloroglucinols which are considered among the most important class of compounds associated with St. John's wort's wound-healing properties. The seed capsules can then be added to the already prepared oil for a few weeks; then strain the oil again.

When preparing the oil, bring a mason jar into the field with you. Fill the jar completely with the herb and cover with your favorite type of oil (olive, wheat germ, etc.). When you get home, pour the oil and herb into a food processor or blender and turn it on for only a few seconds. This should thoroughly masticate the plant, releasing its valuable constituents into the oil. Let this preparation stand for two weeks, occasionally exposing it to direct sun, such as on a window sill for a few hours a day. At the end of two weeks strain the oil and store in amber bottles. You will have made one of the most versatile wound-healing preparations available.

Some herbalists recommend the extraction oil be heated

to 113°F for 10 days or to 158°F for 12 to 24 hours. Each technique will yield a good oil. After the herb has soaked in the oil for the prescribed time, it should turn a deep burgundy red. Then it is ready to be filtered, bottled and stored for future use. The oil can be filtered by pouring through cheesecloth. This usually suffices for removing all plant parts. When storing extracts, label and date them.

Herbalist Michael Moore recommends allowing the flowering tips of the herbs to sit loosely in an opened paper bag for 24 hours before preparing the oil. This, he states, allows the bugs to leave, and eliminates some of the moisture from the flowers, making for a richer hypericin-yielding oil.

Clay poultice: Mix one tablespoon French green clay or betonite clay with an adequate amount of St. John's wort oil to form a thin paste. Spread the paste evenly 1/8-1/4 inch thick onto a piece of gauze or linen and place on the affected part. Leave on overnight, wash off in the morning and follow with an application of St. John's wort oil. This is a specific therapy for neuralgic pains and inflammations such as shingles or herpes.

COMMERCIAL PREPARATIONS

Today there are a number of high-quality preparations readily available from herbalists or health food stores. These include tablets, capsules, tinctures, other liquid extracts, oils and salves. The majority of clear gelatin capsules lose their potency relatively quickly as the surface area of the herb is exposed to air and light, which can significantly reduce the concentration of specific volatile and light-sensitive constituents. Most tablets are prepared from material that has been standardized to a certain percentage of hypericin (usually 0.1-0.3 percent). These will have greater shelf life as tablets are tightly packed, allowing less of the herb to be exposed to air and light.

The relative quality of tinctures, other liquid extracts and oils is generally reflected in the deep burgundy color of the liquid. The red color is a measure of hypericin and pseudohypericin concentration. Generally speaking, the deeper the color, the higher concentration of these components. If the visible pigments have been extracted well, it is usually an indication that other components have also been extracted as well. Alcohol is also a very good preservative; alcohol preparations will maintain their shelf life for at least two years if stored properly.

Conclusion

St. John's wort is taking its place among the most widely used botanical medicines today. When we consider this single herb's great potential as an effective antidepressant or antiviral, we begin to appreciate the immense value botanical medicines have. Americans are quickly learning that the botanical kingdom has a tremendous amount to offer in our quest for health and healing. There are hundreds of commercially available botanical supplements waiting for Americans to discover. St. John's wort is simply the tip of the iceberg. Plants have provided us with our primary source of medicine since the beginning of time and will continue to do so as long as we have the foresight and wisdom to use them.

Appendix

The following charts represent the studies reviewed by Linde, et al., in the *British Medical Journal* in 1996 (see reference #40, page 60).

Chronology of Placebo-controlled Trials		
Trial	**No. of Patients**	**Diagnoses**
Hoffmann, 1979	60	13 psychogenic, 13 climacteric, 14 involution, 10 somatogenic, 10 juvenile depressive patients
Schlich, 1987	49	Mild to moderately severe depression
Schmidt, 1989	40	Neurotic depression and various others
Harrer, 1991	120	Neurotic depression adjustment disorder
Halama, 1991	50	Neurotic depression, adjustment disorder
Osterheider, 1992	47	Moderately severe to severe endogenous, neurotic or reactive depression
Reh, 1992	50	Neurotic depression, adjustment disorder
König, 1993	112	Psychoaffective disorders w/depressed mood
Quandt, 1993	88	Neurotic depression
Lehrl, 1993	50	Neurotic depression, adjustment disorder
Schmidt, 1993	65	Neurotic depression, adjustment disorder
Sommer, 1994	105	Neurotic depression, adjustment disorder
Hänsgen, 1994	72	Major depression
Hübner, 1994	40	Neurotic depression, adjustment disorder

These studies showed that St. John's wort was superior to placebo and as effective as the standard antidepressant listed.

OF SINGLE ST. JOHN'S WORT PREPARATIONS				
Compared treatment	**St. John's wort preparation**	**Total hypericin (mg/day)**	**Extract (mg/day)**	**Duration (weeks)**
Placebo	Hyperforat	0.6	NA	6
Placebo	Psychotonin M	0.5	350	4
Placebo	Psychotonin M	0.75	500	4
Placebo	Psychotonin M	0.75	500	6
Placebo	Jarsin	1.08	900	4
Placebo	Psychotonin M	0.75	500	8
Placebo	Neuroplant	1	500	8
Placebo	Extract Z 90017	1.00-2.00	500-1000	6
Placebo	Psychotonin M	0.75	500	4
Placebo	Jarsin	1.08	900	4
Placebo	Jarsin	1.08	900	6
Placebo	Jarsin 300	2.7	900	4
Placebo	Jarsin 300	2.7	900	4
Placebo	Jarsin 300	2.7	900	4

CHRONOLOGY OF TRIALS COMPARING SINGLE ST. JOHN'S

Trial	No. of Patients	Diagnoses
Warnecke, 1986	60	Climacteric (endogenous, involutive, reactive) depressive patients
Werth, 1989	30	Reactive depression after informing patients of necessity of amputation
Kugler, 1990	80	Mild to moderately severe depressions (endogenous depression excluded)
Bergmann, 1993	80	Single and recurrent mild and moderate severe depression episodes
Vorbach, 1994	135	Major depression, neurotic depression, adjustment disorders
Harrer, 1994	102	Single moderately severe depressive episode

DSM-III-R = Diagnostic criteria for major depression.
HDS = Hamilton Depression Scale;
DS = depression scale; DSI depression status inventory;
ICD 9 & 10 = International Classification of Depression;
BfS = Befindlichkeits-Skala (von Zerssen, adjective mood scale).

Wort Preparations with Conventional Antidepressants				
Compared treatment	**St. John's wort preparation**	**Total hypericin (mg/day)**	**Extract (mg/day)**	**Duration (wks)**
Diazepam 6 mg	Hyperforat	0.4	NA	12
Imipramine 50 mg	Psychotonin M	0.75	500	2
Bromazepam 6 mg	Psychotonin M	0.75	500	4
Amitriptyline 30 mg	Esbericum	0.75	NA	6
Imipramine	Jarsin 300	2.7	900	6
Maprotiline 75 mg	Jarsin 300	2.7	900	4

PROFILE OF THE PRIMARY *HYPERICUM* PREPARATIONS USED IN THE DEPRESSION STUDIES REVIEWED IN THE *BMJ* ARTICLE (Upton, et al., 1997)		
Preparation Name	**Total Extract/day**	**Total Hypericin/day**
Esbericum	i.v.	0.75 mg
Extract Z 90017	500-1000 mg	1-2 mg
Hyperforat	i.v.	0.4-0.6 mg
Jarsin (tablets)	900 mg	1.08 mg
Jarsin 300 (tablets) [LI 160]	900 mg	2.7 mg
Neurapas	600 mg	0.48 mg
Neuroplant (caps)	500 mg	1 mg
Psychotonin M® (drops)	350-500 mg	0.5-0.75 mg
Sedariston*	300-600 mg	0.45-0.9 mg

*Also contains valerian extract

Chemical Constituents of St. John's Wort

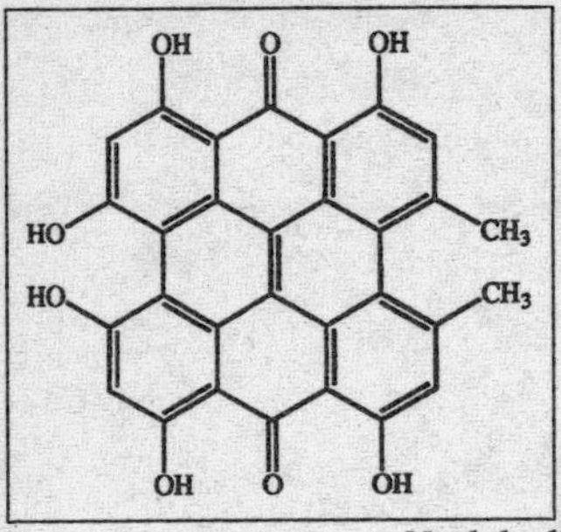

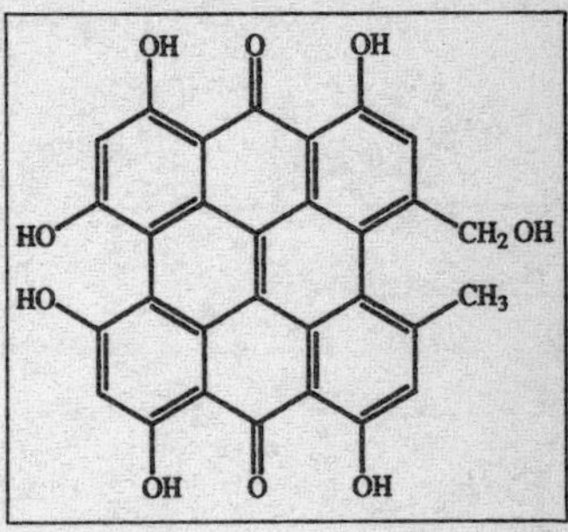

Naphthodianthrones

Hypericin (0.02-2.5%)

Pseudohypericin (ca. 0.04-3.6%)

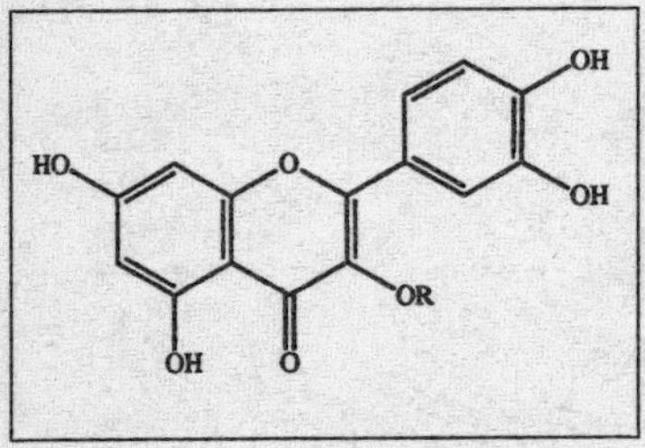

Flavonol Glycosides (2-4%)

R = H	Quercetin
R = a-l-rhamnosyl	Quercetrin
R = ß-D-glucosyl	Isoquercetrin
R = ß-D-galactosyl	Hyperoside
R = ß-rutinosyl	Rutin

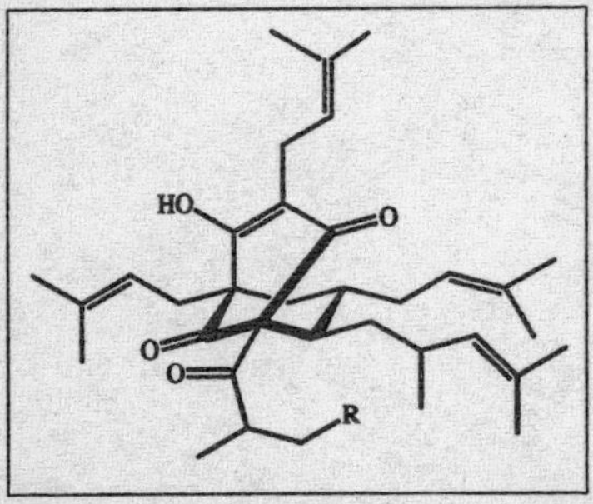

Phloroglucinols

R = H: Hyperforin (2.0-4.5%)

R = CH_3: Adhyperforin (0.2-1.9%)

References

1. Pratt, A. *Wild Flowers*. London: Society for Promoting Christian Knowledge; 1853.
2. Vickery, A.R. Traditional uses and folklore of *Hypericum* in the British Isles. *Economic Botany*. 1981; 289-295.
3. Hobbs, C. St. John's wort: *Hypericum perforatum* L. A review. *HerbalGram*. 1989; 18/19:24-33.
4. Riddle, J. Dioscorides on Medicine and Pharmacy. University of Texas Press, 1985.
5. Berghöfer, R., Hölzl, J. Isolation of 13,' II8-biapigenin (amentoflavone) from *Hypericum perforatum. Planta Medica*. 1989; 91.
6. Nahrstedt, A., Butterweck, V. Biologically active and other chemical constituents of the herb of *Hypericum perforatum L. Pharmacopsychiatry*. 1997 (in press).
7. Melzer, R., Fricke, U., Hölzl, J., Podehl, R., Zylka, J. Procyanidins from *Hypericum perforatum:* effects on isolated guinea pig hearts. *Planta Medica*. 1989; 55:655-656.
8. Gurevich, A.I., Dobrynin, V.N., Kolosov, M.N., et al. Hyperforin, an antibiotic from *Hypericum perforatum. Chem. Abstracts*. 1971; 75:95625t. *Antibiotiki (Moscow)*. 971; 16:510-513.
9. Suzuki, O., Katsumata, Y., Oya, M., Chari, V.M., Vermes, B., Wagner, H., Hostettmann, K. Inhibition of type-A and type-B monoamine oxidases by naturally occurring xanthones. *Planta Medica*. 42; 1981: 17-21.
10. Rocha, L., Marston, A., Auxiliadora, M., et al. An antifungal g-pyrone and xanthones with monoamine oxidase inhibitory activity from *Hypericum brasiliense. Phytochemistry*. 1994; 36.
11. Suzuki, O., Katsumata, Y., Oya, M., Bladt, S., Wagner, H. Inhibition of monoamine oxidase by hypericin. *Planta Medica*. 1984; 50:272-274.

12. Demisch, L., Hölzl, J., Golnik, B., Kacynarczyk. Identification of MAO type-A inhibitors in *Hypericum perforatum* L. (Hyperforat™). *Pharmacopsychiatry.* 1989; 22:194.
13. Sparenberg, B., Demisch, L. Hölzl, J. Antidepressive constituents of St. John's wort. *Chem. Abstracts.* 1993; 119:85914z. *PZ Wiss.* 1993; 6:50-54.
14. Bladt, S., Wagner, H. Inhibition of MAO by fractions and constituents of *Hypericum* extract. *J. Geriatric Psychiatry Neurology.* 1994; 7:S57-59.
15. Höltje, H.D., Walper, A. Molecular modeling of the antidepressive mechanism of *Hypericum* ingredients. *Nervenheilkunde.* 1993; 12:339-340.
16. Thiede, H.M., Walper, A. Inhibition of MAO and COMT by *Hypericum* extracts and hypericin. *J. Geriatric Psychiatry Neurology.* 1994; 7:S34-38.
17. Upton, R., Cott, J., Graff, A., Williamson, E., Bunting, D., Gatherum, D., Walker, E., et al, Monograph: St. John's Wort. American Herbal Pharmacopoeia; *Herbal Gram* American Botanical Council, Austin 1997.
18. Lieberman, H.R., Waldhauser, F., Garfield, G., Lynch, H., Wurtman, R. Effects of melatonin on human mood and performance. *Brain Research* 323, 201-207, 1984.
19. Demisch, L., Nispel, J., Sielaff, T., Gebhart, P., Koehler, C. Influences of nocturnal light pulses of different intensities on melatonin secretions before and after subchronic administration of Hyperforat™ in healthy volunteers. *Pharmacopsychiatry,* 1997.
20. Harrer, G., Hübner, W.D., Podzuweit, H. Effectiveness and tolerance of the *Hypericum* extract LI 160 in comparison with imipramine: randomized double-blind study with 135 outpatients. *J. Geriatric Psychiatry Neurology.* 1994; 7:S24-28.
21. Wölk, H., Burkard, G., Grünwald, J. Benefits and risks of the *Hypericum* extract LI 160: drug-monitoring study with 3250 patients. *J. Geriatric Psychiatry Neurology.* 1994; 7:S34-38.

22. Sommer, H., Harrer, G. Placebo-controlled double-blind study examining the effectiveness of a *Hypericum* preparation in 105 mildly depressed patients. *J. Geriatric Psychiatry Neurology*. 1994; 7:S9-11.
23. Murray, M., Pizzorno, J. Encyclopedia of Natural Healing, Prima Publishing, Rocklin, CA 1991.
24. Meruelo, D., Lavie, G., Lavie, D. Therapeutic agents with dramatic antiretroviral activity and little toxicity at effective doses: aromatic polycyclic diones hypericin and pseudohypericin. *Proc. Natl. Acad. Sci. USA*. 1988; 85:5230-5234.
25. Takahashi, I., Nakanishi, S., Kobayashi, E., Nakano, H., Suzuki, K., Tamaoki, T. Hypericin and pseudohypericin specifically inhibit protein kinase C: possible relation to their antiretroviral activity. *Biochem. Biophys. Res. Comm.* 1989; 165:1207-1212.
26. Lavie, G., Valentine, F., Levin, B., et al. Studies of the mechanisms of the antiretroviral agents hypericin and pseudohypericin. *Proc. Natl. Acad. Sci.* 1989; 86:5963-5967.
27. Priest, A.W., Priest, L.R. Herbal Medication. London: L.N. Fowler & Co. Ltd.; 1982.
28. Liske, E., Wüstenberg, P., Kohnen, R. Relief for psychovegetative symptoms during menopause: A new herbal combination of St. John's wort and black cohosh. *2nd International Congress on Phytomedicine*. Munich; 1996: SL-90.
29. Gaind, K.N., Ganjoo, T.N. Antibacterial principle of *Hypericum perforatum* Linn. *Indian J. Pharm.* 1959; 21:172-175.
30. Khosa, R.L., Bhatia, N. Antifungal effect of *Hypericum perforatum* Linn. *J. Sci. Res. Plants Med.* 1982; 3:49-50.
31. Shakirova, K.K., Garagulya, A.D., Khazanovich, R.L. Antimicrobial properties of some species of St. John's wort cultivated in Uzbekistan. *Mikrobiol. Zh.* 1970; 32:494-497.
32. Negrash, A.K., Pochinok, P.Y. Comparative study of chemotherapeutic and pharmacological properties of antimicrobial preparations from common St. John's wort. *Fitontsidy, Mater. Seveshch.* 1972; 6th meeting: 198-200.

33. Saljic, J. Ointment for the treatment of burns. Ger. Offen. 1975; 2:406-452. *Chem. Abstracts*. 1975; 197797h.
34. Rao, S.G., Laxminarayana, A.U., Saraswathi, L.U., Padma, G.M., Ganesh, R., Kulkarni, D.R. *Calendula* and *Hypericum*: two homeopathic drugs promoting wound healing in rats. *Fitoterapia*. 1991; 6:508-510.
35. Krylov, A.A., Ibatov, A.N. The use of an infusion of St. John's wort in the combined treatment of alcoholics with peptic ulcer and chronic gastritis. *Vrach-Delo*. 1993; Feb-Mar (2-3): 146-148.
36. Hahn, G. *Hypericum perforatum* (St. John's wort) - a medicinal herb used in antiquity and still of interest today. *Journal of Naturopathic Medicine*. 1992; 3:94-96.
37. Vogel, H.C.A. *The Nature Doctor*. Mainstream Publishing. Edinburgh, 1990.
38. Weiss, R.F., Meuss, A.R. (trans.). *Herbal Medicine*. Arcanum: Beaconsfield Publishers Ltd.; 1988.
39. Schulz, H., Jobert, M. Effects of *Hypericum* extract on the sleep EEG in older volunteers. *J. Geriatric Psychiatry Neurology*. 1994; 7:S39-43.
40. Linde, K., Ramirez, G., Mulrow, C.D., Pauls, A., Weidenhammer, W., Melchart, D. St. John's wort for depression an overview and meta-analysis of randomized clinical trials. *British Medical Journal*. 1996; 313:253-258.
41. DAC. Deutscher Arzneimittel-Codex. 3rd Supplement 91 ed.; 1986.
42. ESCOP. Monograph St. John's wort. European Scientific Cooperative for Phytomedicines. The Netherlands: Meppel; 1996.
43. Moore, M. Medicinal Plants of the Pacific West. Red Crane Books, Santa Fe. 1993.

Resources

Bibliography

Blumenthal, M., Grünwald, J., Hall, T., Riggins, C.W., Rister, R.S. (Eds.); Klein, S., Rister, R.S. (trans.). German Commission E Monographs: Therapeutic Monographs of Medicinal Plants for Human Use. Austin, TX: American Botanical Council; 1997 (in press).

Bombardelli, E., Morazzoni, P. *Hypericum perforatum. Fitoterapia.* 1995; 66:43-68.

ESCOP. Monograph on St. John's wort. European Scientific Cooperative for Phytomedicines. The Netherlands: Meppel; 1996.

Felter, H.W. *Eclectic Materia Medica, Pharmacology and Therpaeutics.* : John K. Scudder; 1922.

Gerard, J. *The Herbal.* Revised and enlarged by T. Johnson. New York: Reprinted by Dover Publications Inc. (1975); 1633.

King, J. *The American Dispensatory* 7th ed. Cincinnati: Moore, Wilstach & Baldwin; 1866.

Leuschner, J. Preclinical toxicological profile of *Hypericum* extract LI 160. *2nd International Congress on Phytomedicine.* Munich; 1996.

McGuffin, M., Hobbs, C., Upton, R., Goldberg, *A. Botanical Safety Handbook.* Boca Raton: CRC Press; 1997 (in press).

Nahrstedt, A., Butterweck, V. Biologically active and other chemical constituents of the herb of *Hypericum perforatum* L. *Pharmacopsychiatry.* 1997 (in press).

Pharmacopoeia Helvetica. Monograph on St. John's wort; 1996.

Vorbach, E.U., Hübner, W.D., Arnoldt, K.H. Effectiveness and tolerance of the *Hypericum* extract LI 160 in comparison with imipramine: randomized double-blind study with 135 outpatients. *J. Geriatric Psychiatry Neurology.* 1994; 7:S19-23.

RECOMMENDED READING

Feeling Good Handbook by David Burns. New York: William Morrow, 1989.

Immune Power by Jon Kaiser. New York: St. Martin's Press,1995.

Hypericum Monograph: American Herbal Pharmacopoeia, Upton et al, Austin, Texas: American Botanical Council, 1997.

Hypericum: Literature review by Christopher Hobbs, *HerbalGram*, Austin, Texas: American Botanical Council, 1989.

Hypericum & Depression by Harold Bloomfield, Michael Nordfors, Peter Williams. Los Angeles: Prelude Press, 1997.

How to Heal Depression by Harold Bloomfield, Michael Nordfors, Peter Williams. Los Angeles: Prelude Press, 1995.

Index